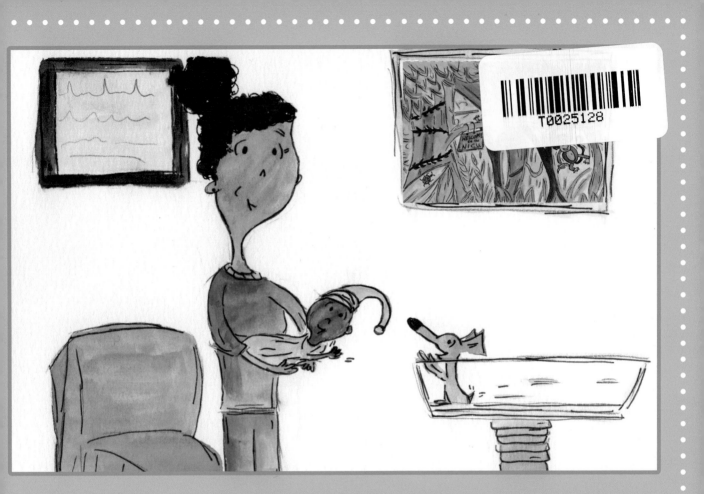

Hi there and welcome to the neonatal intensive care unit –
the NICU!
When I was born, I had to spend some time here.
As do a whole lot of babies.

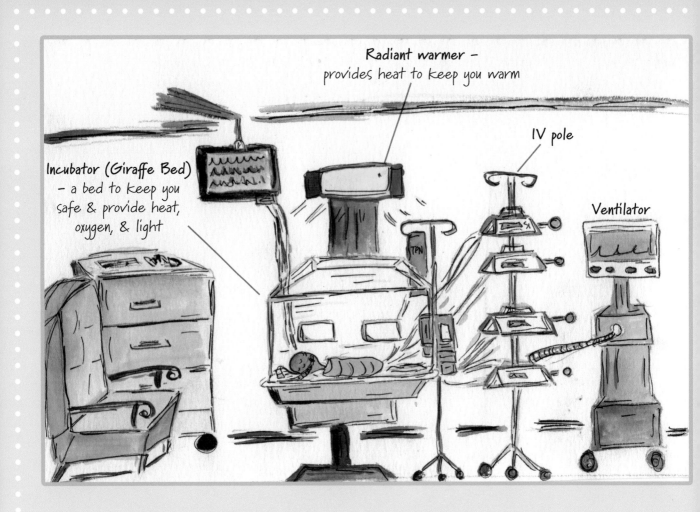

Radiant warmer – provides heat to keep you warm

IV pole

Incubator (Giraffe Bed) – a bed to keep you safe & provide heat, oxygen, & light

Ventilator

It is a special place that offers special care for situations like being born too early, having your intestines outside your belly (what!), and so many other things.

Look around. It will seem overwhelming at first.

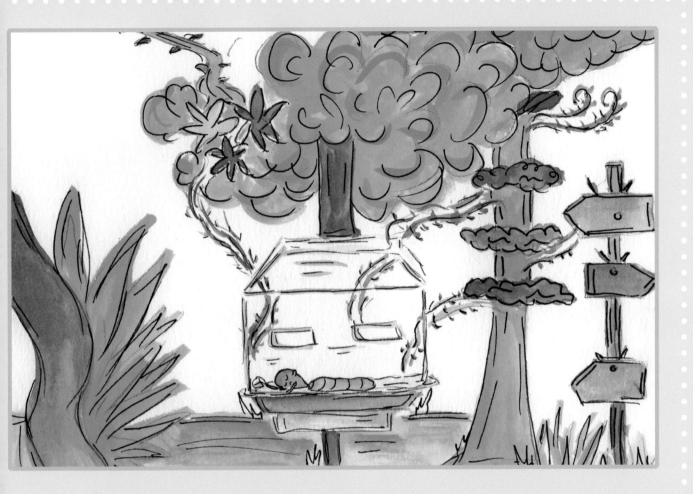

And to me, it even seemed more like a jungle
than a hospital unit! All the machines. All the devices.
Lines, tubes… Oh my!

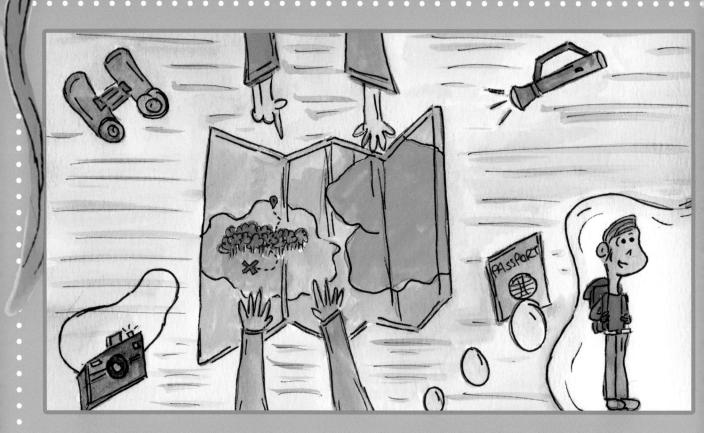

Now my parents knew I was going to be in the NICU before I was born because my mom had a prenatal ultrasound that showed I would need special help. So they were able to plan — like planning a trip to the jungle.

But there were still surprises — no matter how much they prepared. Other parents might crash-land in this jungle right after you are born. An unexpected trip to the NICU without any preparation. That might be a little scarier.

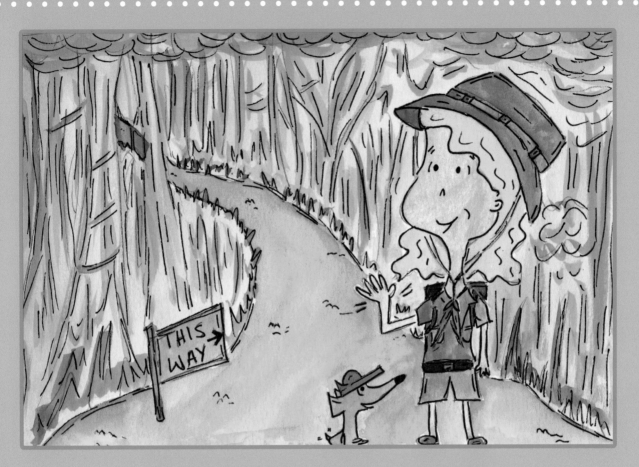

Whichever way you get to the NICU –
planned, or unplanned, it's helpful to have a guide.
And luckily, the NICU is filled with guides! Guides that include
doctors, surgeons, nurses, therapists, and so many more people.
They have many jobs to help take care of you. Like when your
family can't be with you, they spend time with you. The nurses
are particularly good at it!

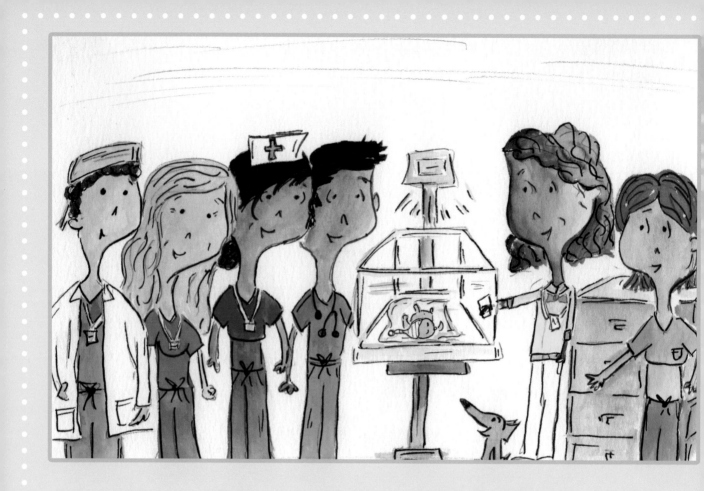

So, when my mom or dad has to go home to be with my
sibilings, they know I'm still in extra good hands!

These guides will also let your family know when
you're too small or fragile to be held.
But don't worry, we still know you're here next to us!

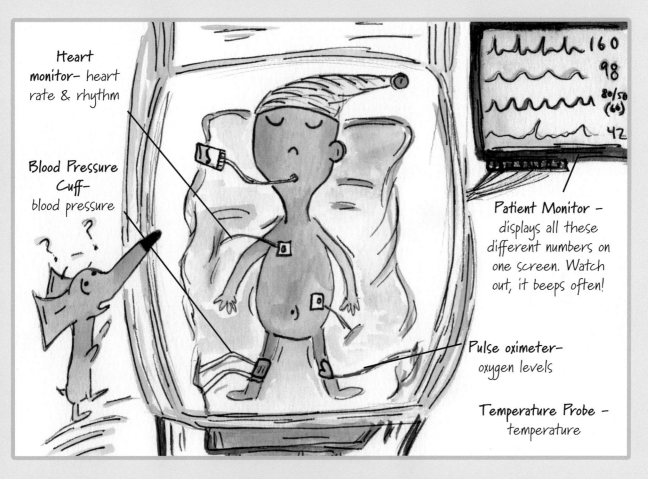

All the Cords

So let me teach you about some of the things in the NICU.
Once you become familiar with them, they will be less scary.
Let's start with the cords that you'll have
plugged into you and what they measure.
You're like a phone being charged!

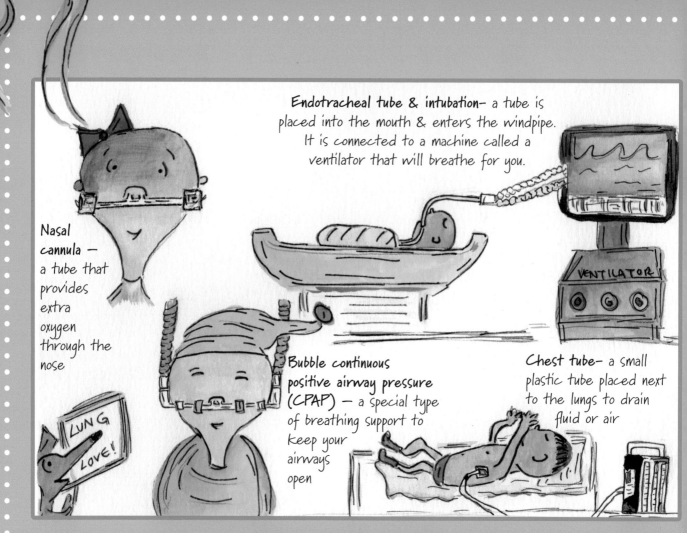

Nasal cannula — a tube that provides extra oxygen through the nose

Endotracheal tube & intubation- a tube is placed into the mouth & enters the windpipe. It is connected to a machine called a ventilator that will breathe for you.

VENTILATOR

Bubble continuous positive airway pressure (CPAP) — a special type of breathing support to keep your airways open

Chest tube- a small plastic tube placed next to the lungs to drain fluid or air

LUNG LOVE!

Lung Love!

Breathing is, of course, important. Some babies need lots of help breathing. Some only need a little. Respiratory therapists are our breathing guides. They can teach you about all the different devices because they're in charge of them!

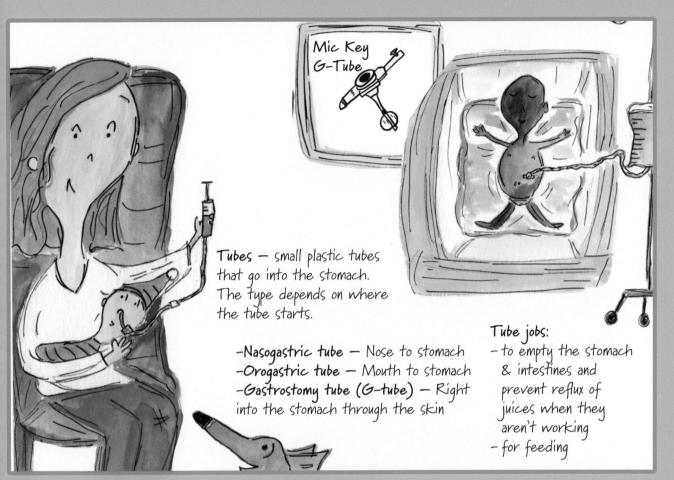

Mic Key G-Tube

Tubes — small plastic tubes that go into the stomach. The type depends on where the tube starts.

- Nasogastric tube — Nose to stomach
- Orogastric tube — Mouth to stomach
- Gastrostomy tube (G-tube) — Right into the stomach through the skin

Tube jobs:
- to empty the stomach & intestines and prevent reflux of juices when they aren't working
- for feeding

FOOD!

What about food you say? Food is also important! Some babies are not ready to eat so they get special nutrition through their veins (called TPN). Other babies might have tubes that go into their bellies. If you're ready to start eating by mouth, your speech therapist guide and lactation consultant will help!

Broviac central venous line (CVL) — a short IV that goes from the neck, groin, or under the collarbone to the heart

CVL

PICC

PICC — a long IV that goes from the arms or legs all the way to the heart

Umbilical catheter — an IV that goes into the umbilical cord blood vessels

Arterial line — an IV that goes into an artery (instead of a vein) to measure blood pressure

IVs upon IVs...

Ok. So you're sick of all the IV lines. I was too. But it helped to know about them. IVs are used for antibiotics, medicines, fluids, and/or IV food (TPN). And our nurses help keep them from being a knot of tangled spaghetti.

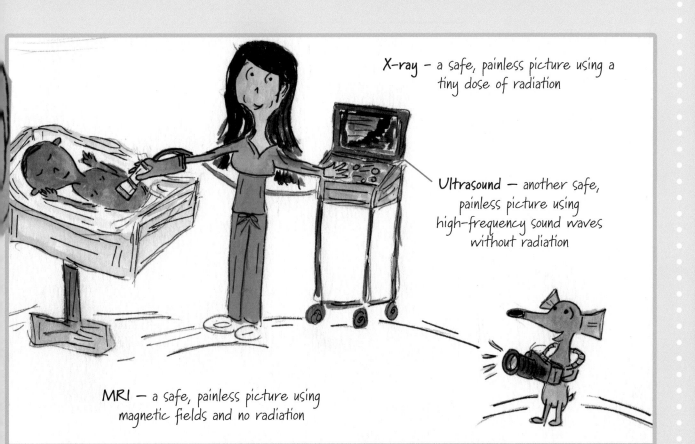

X-ray – a safe, painless picture using a tiny dose of radiation

Ultrasound — another safe, painless picture using high-frequency sound waves without radiation

MRI — a safe, painless picture using magnetic fields and no radiation

Say cheese!
It's picture time!
Sometimes we need X-rays, ultrasounds, or MRIs.
These are safe, painless ways to take pictures of our insides with little to no radiation.

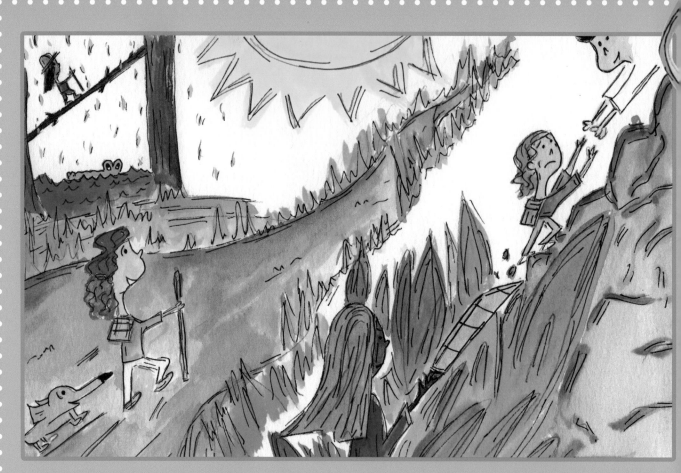

So now that you know a little more, you also need to know that not every path through the NICU is easy. And everyone's path is different – just like paths through a jungle. Some paths are long and seem never-ending. Some are short. Some are filled with sunlight. Others with torrential rain. Some paths are wide open. Some are overgrown with brush. Some paths you must hack your way through. However, each path is special.

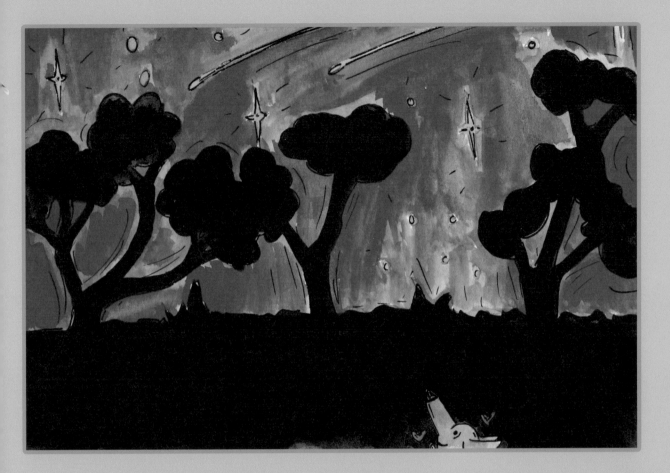

And just like jungle plants, us babies grow and change. Some of us will grow big and strong quickly. Some may start slow and weak and then flourish after time. Others may not survive and instead become never-forgotten heroes – shining like stars in the jungle sky.

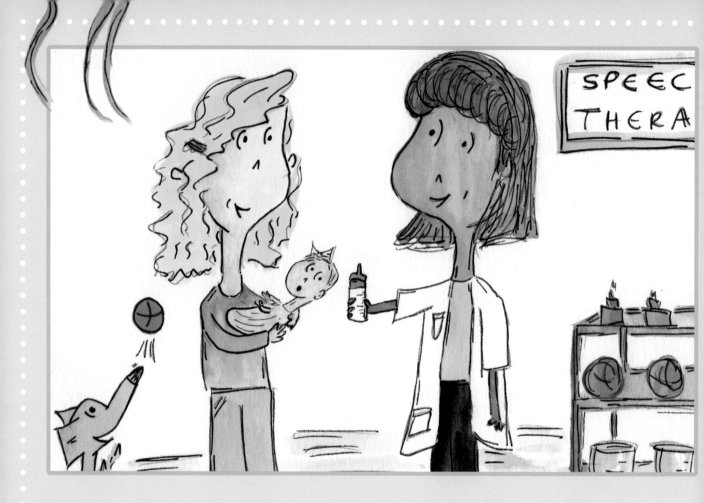

Someday, you may graduate out of the NICU. Some of your guides may stay in touch and continue to help you. Or you may see them at NICU reunions, annual picnics, or even the grocery store!

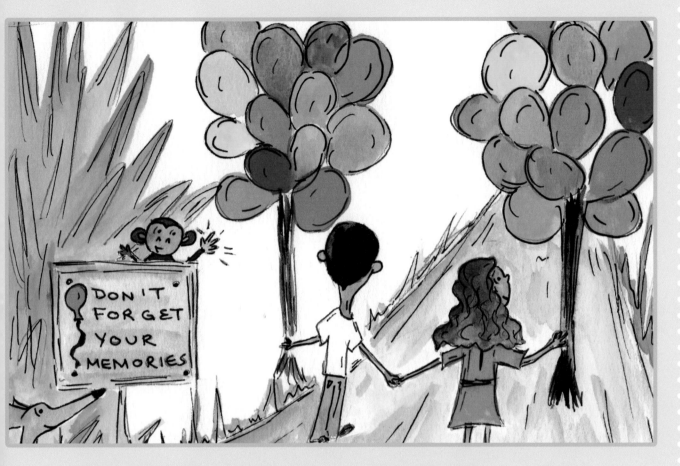

You won't remember your time in the NICU, but your parents will. They will have reminders of that time – just like memories from a jungle adventure.
Good memories and bad ones.
Exciting milestones and rock bottoms.

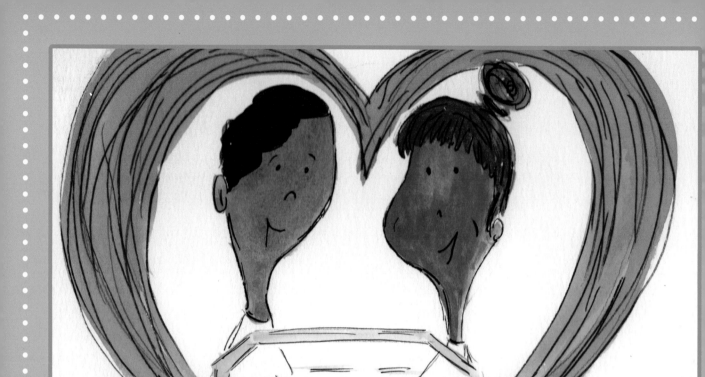

These memories are all part of your special NICU story.

Common NICU Procedures

Neonatologists are your primary guides in charge of these procedures. They'll call other guides, like **pediatric** surgeons, to help with special things.

Here are some of the common NICU procedures:

– **Intubation** – placing a tube into the mouth, down to the lungs. This connects to a ventilator to help you breathe.

– **Line placement** – special IVs need to be placed in radiology or sometimes in the operating room (Central venous line).

– **Feeding tube placement** – this can be a tube in your nose, mouth, or right into your stomach (G-tube). A G-tube is put in surgically in the operating room.

– **Chest tube placement** – this is a small tube that drains fluid or air from around your lungs.

– **Phototherapy** – use of special light to treat newborn jaundice (caused by high bilirubin levels!)

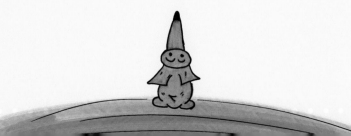

NICU Diagnoses

1. Prematurity
2. Intrauterine growth restriction (IUGR)
3. Cardiac (Heart)
   a. Ventral or atrial septal defect (VSD, ASD)
   b. Patent Ductus Arteriosus (PDA)
   c. Coarctation of the aorta
   d. Tetralogy of Fallot
   e. Transposition of the great arteries
4. Gastrointestinal (Stomach, Intestines)
   a. Feeding issues
   b. Spontaneous Intestinal Perforation (SIP)
   c. Necrotizing enterocolitis (NEC)
   d. Gastroschisis
   e. Omphalocele
5. Neurologic (Brain)
   a. Intraventricular hemorrhage (IVH)
   b. Hypoxic Ischemic Encephalopathy
   c. Seizure
   d. Stroke
6. Hematology (Blood)
   a. Jaundice
   b. Anemia
7. Respiratory (Lungs)
   a. Respiratory distress syndrome
   b. Transient Tachypnea of Newborn
   c. Apnea of prematurity
   d. Bronchopulmonary dysplasia
   e. Persistent pulmonary hypertension of the newborn (PPHN)
   f. Tracheoesophageal fistula
   g. Congenital diaphragmatic hernia

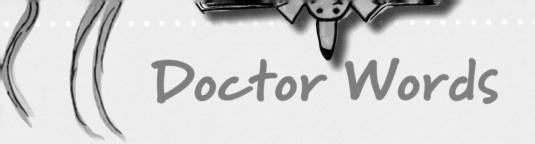

Doctor Words

Jaundice – When skin & eyes turn a yellow color. This is from high bilirubin levels which is common in newborns. It is treated with a special light therapy called phototherapy.

Intraventricular hemorrhage (IVH) — Bleeding into a part of the brain (the ventricles). It is common in premature babies. We don't know what causes it.

Apnea – Pauses in breathing. Nurses will rub our backs to remind us to breathe. Apnea is common in newborns. It tends to go away as we grow.

Bradycardia – A slow heart rate (or pulse). Sometimes this is caused by apnea episodes.

Vasopressors – Special IV medicines used to increase blood pressure when it's low.

Replogle – A special tube that goes into your mouth or nose to empty the stomach and intestines and prevent reflux of juices when there is a blockage or they aren't working.

ECMO - (Extracorporeal-outside the body, Membrane-artificial lung, Oxygenation-giving your body oxygen): A temporary machine that takes your blood, oxygenates it, and returns it to you. This normally is the job of the lungs but when the lungs need to rest, ECMO can do the work.

TPN – Total parenteral nutrition. Nutrition given through an IV when we can't eat by mouth. It supplies all daily nutritional requirements.

Prematurity - Being born early (before 37 weeks). This is the most common reason for needing NICU care.

Meet the Author:
Dr. Maria Baimas-George

Maria Baimas-George MD MPH is a surgeon, training to specialize in abdominal transplantation. Inspired by her patients and mentors, she writes and illustrates books explaining medical and surgical conditions to children and their loved ones. Her goal is to create books that provide useful information to help with understanding and to offer comfort and hope.

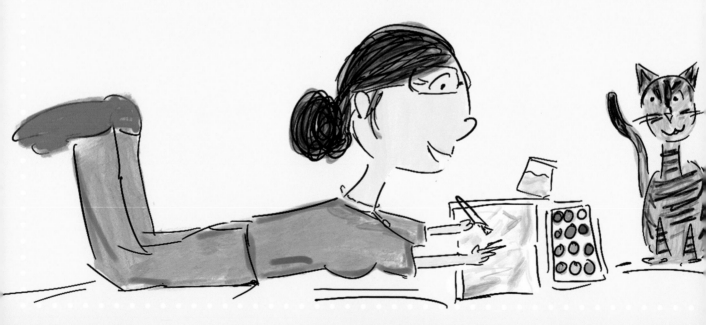